WEIGHT LOSS

A Practical, Step-By-Step Guide for Natural Weight Loss

Lose weight easily and quickly by understanding the 3 main factors that will shed off those pounds

JULIA RAY

I0428201

Table Of Contents

Introduction

Welcome reader!

I just want to say a huge thank you and congratulate you for purchasing the book, "Weight Loss". In this book, you will be able to find the easiest ways to lose over ten pounds in JUST one week, sounds crazy right?

This book contains proven steps and strategies on how to lose one stone of body fat in one week, just by following the steps (including dieting) provided later on in this book for a successful and shocking result. AND EVEN MORE...! Not only does this book contain information for dieting, but also includes:

- A   recipe   guide   for   the   5   healthiest   meals   (How   To   Make   Them)
- Workout routines (Exercises Done At Home) and much more...

Feeling interested? Well, you have purchased the right book and I promise that you will not regret spending a few coins for a book that would be worth quite a fortune. So you ask, "How is it possible to lose over ten pounds in one week and if so, what must I do in order to achieve such a great transformation in a short period of time?" Well, that's exactly what you will be learning step-by-step in this book. Thanks once again for purchasing this book.

Sit back, relax and I hope you enjoy it!

Chapter One: Weight Loss – An Overview

Fad diets, exercise ticks and quick methods to lose weight – you've starved yourself, only to finally decide that it isn't worth it and thrown your hands up in the air, because this is just not working. But the truth is that weight loss doesn't have to be that difficult; in fact, it can be the easiest thing in the world, if you know what you're doing.

Weight loss, in simple terms, is simply shedding those excess pounds that seem to consistently float around your body. Medically, it's defined as the decrease in weight due to a drop in bodily fluid, fat or muscle mass. Each body has a particular ideal weight, dependent on a number of factors such as your height and your age, and it's best to hover close to this ideal weight to live longer, happier and healthier!

Why should you think about losing weight? For most people, it's about fitting into those skinny jeans, which is perfectly fine, but we tend to overlook the actual health benefits of losing weight. Check out some of the medical reasons for you to lose weight –

- Avoid Type 2 Diabetes or a Pre-Diabetic situation. When you're overweight, your cells find it harder to respond to insulin, since the extra fat acts as a barrier. This means that your rotating blood sugar levels are high in your body and your pancreas, having to push excess insulin, will say *'I'm done!'* after a point of time, leading to diabetes.
- Avoid heart diseases. Being overweight exposes you to higher blood pressure and cholesterol levels, which definitely could cause heart problems.
- Get rid of pain-free joints and keep your mobility even in old age. When you're overweight, your joints take a beating because they're bearing more pressure.
- Improve your energy levels; despite popular belief, exercising makes you feel *more* awake instead of tiring you out!

The advantages to losing weight aren't just physical. The psychological benefits are just as powerful! Research has shown that shedding those excess pounds results in higher self-confidence levels and a much lower rate of depression – obviously, when you look and feel fabulous, any anxiety you have will fade away and you will be more confident in life! Additionally, exercising releases endorphins, which help you feel good – exercise and depression have a cause and effect relationship with one another. You exercise to rid yourself of depression, and once you start losing pounds, you feel more energized (when you're depressed, you have zero energy) and you step your workout more, lose more weight and then the cycle continues!

But then the opposite is true as well; a lot of people fall into depression because they aren't able to lose weight. This, though, is not so much a fault of their body, as they take to it be, as it is the diet and the exercise patterns they follow. The biggest mistake most people make is assuming that working towards losing weight is temporary – it's *not*.

People generally want to go on a few week diets, lose a couple of pounds and then go back to their old lifestyle of eating junk and not exercising. It's like a break from your routine to get something done and then returning to your routine. Logically, how can you expect that to sustain the weight loss you achieved over the few weeks, if you don't *maintain* the same routine?

In essence, sustained weight loss and management doesn't mean just going on a crash diet – it's *lifestyle* change. And those words are very easy to throw around, but believe me, it's the hardest thing you'll ever do, which is why it's so difficult to lose weight and then maintain it. You need make weight loss a part of your *daily* routine, instead of 'taking time out'; even after your diet is done, you need to make healthy food choices and continue to keep to those choices instead of shifting back to your old eating habits.

What you should do, then, is use the ideas given in this book as a kick-starter to your new lifestyle. The one-week plan? Make it your first step into a healthier life; think of it, not as something you have to get through, but the beginning. Your attitude at the end of it should be – *hey, look, I've finished one whole week of this kind of a lifestyle, let me continue and make it an instinct instead of 'taking time to diet'!*

Chapter Two – Pre-Requisite Lifestyle Changes for Weight Loss

The problem with weight loss, as I keep saying, is that it's taken in isolation – it isn't just about losing pounds quickly, it's about maintaining it.

Let me ask you a question – how many people do you know indulge in that extra fatty, extra delicious brownie after lunch, simply because they've completed a good cardio in the morning? Or how many times have you yourself managed to skip workout with the excuse that you're too tired or that you don't have time? The fact is, we want to lose weight, but we don't want to make the changes that are necessary for it.

That brownie you wanted to eat because you worked out? It adds more calories than you burned today. You may be too tired to work out, but you can make sure you keep your day filled with activity – instead of driving to work, walk instead, so that you still get your workout for the day.

You see how easily we make excuses when it comes to weight loss management and maintenance. We need to change our lifestyles instead of working out fad diets – for example, if you haven't exercised regularly before, start now. You don't have to go to the gym each day, instead just shift daily practices to be healthier. Walk to your work or if you're at home, do 10 Jumping Jacks while you watch TV. The trick isn't to take time out for it and just 'be done with it'; it's to make it a part of your daily routine so it doesn't seem too hard.

Before we jump into the whole gamut of *'how do I lose weight?'*, let's first understand what's happening in your body. The thing about weight loss is that different people have different body types and a weight loss program has to be highly individualistic to suit your needs. Why you're overweight is something only *you* can figure out – for instance, for a lot of women, issues like PCOS or hypothyroidism is a major cause for weight gain. This means that every weight loss program you look at can only be a *guideline* for you to start your own, personalized plan to fix your health.

However, despite that, there are certain generic things you can keep an eye on, some things that are common to every person, regardless of your medical issues. Exercising every day, for example, is something that is a must for everyone – *what* exercise you do may differ according to your specific condition, but exercising in general is necessary.

So when it comes to a daily routine of weight loss, these are some of the things we need to keep in mind –

Food

I will not say 'diet'; that term, in my personal opinion, is the bane of weight loss, because diets are generally temporary and imply a break from routine. Our goal is the opposite – you need to make *weight loss* your routine, so instead of going on a one-week 'diet', we will look at a one-week *meal plan* that'll help you start your new lifestyle. We'll take a look at some easy-to-make healthy recipes and then you can slowly make the shift from junk food to a food pattern that keeps you fit!

Essentially, the best foods that help with weight loss are those that help boost your metabolism, as well as keep you energetic for a long time so that you don't feel hungry and overeat. That means eating a lot of proteins, high fibers and even a few good fats – it's *carbs* that you need to avoid, along with those extra starch and sugar contents.

Exercising

The most important thing when it comes to weight loss, other than food, is exercise. For any kind of a healthy lifestyle, you need to work out daily. Exercise makes a difference to both physical and mental health – physically, it takes away those extra pounds and helps you remain fit.

When you exercise, your body releases endorphins, the purpose of which is to reduce the perception of pain in your muscles as you work out. But an added effect of these is that you feel happy – endorphins are feel-good hormones. This is why exercise is often used as a clinical method of treating depression and anxiety – it's a natural way to fight these issues.

Counting Calories

Assuming an average situation, without the complications of medical issues such as hypothyroidism or PCOS, the best way to bring your weight down is count your calories. If your goal is to build your body and muscle stature, then this becomes even more important! There are two main things to remember when it comes counting calories and weight loss – calorie surplus and calorie deficit.

Surplus is easy to understand – this is when you consume more calories in a day than you burn, which leads to an increase in weight in the form of muscle or fat. If you're a body builder, for instance, you may require a calorie surplus to help improve muscle definition, or you could simply want to put on weight since you're too skinny. In either case, allowing yourself a surplus doesn't mean randomly stuffing things down your throat – this is a *planned* calorie intake, so you need to consult your nutrition and figure out the healthy way of eating more.

For weight loss, it's calorie deficit you need to focus on. In simple terms, this means eating lesser calories that what your body burns to give you energy; or, you burn more calories through exercise than what you consume. Ultimately, it means that your body doesn't have the calories it needs to do its daily tasks – there's a deficit in your system, which your body makes for by burning the stored fat. This is why you lose pounds when you eat less – your body is using the excess, stored fat to do the daily jobs it needs to.

Now the problem with calorie deficit is that people assume it means you starve yourself – that's wrong! When you starve yourself, you end up overeating and adding more pounds; your body needs nourishment, so any food you eat, it'll *store* instead of burning, since you're not feeding it regularly.

So what you need to do is plan a calorie deficit that suits your body – you can't do too much, or you'll gain weight instead of losing it. Studies show that a 20% deficit is best for an average weight loss program; that means that if your body is accustomed to consuming 2000 calories in a day, you need to reduce 20% of that consumption, which is 400 calories – so you eat only 1600 calories in the day and your body burns another 400 calories from your stored fat to make up for the deficit.

You have to be *extremely* careful while planning this; exercise and calorie counting can definitely help you shed pounds, but you need to make sure you don't burn yourself out doing it. A moderate calorie deficit is good, just as a moderate exercise plan is what you need.

Sleep

According to the Centre for Disease Control and Prevention, more than 35% of people in the USA are sleep deprived. I know it seems counter-productive – you want to move more and eat less to lose weight, but now I'm telling you to sleep! Research tells us that if you don't sleep enough, you experience a 55% reduction in the amount of weight you lose. That's more than half of your effort going down the drain!

The logic behind it is simple. Insulin is the hormone that helps your body decide where and when to store fat; if you don't sleep at night, your body loses its ability to use that insulin properly. Like with the diabetes situation, your cells turn insulin resistant – excess insulin is secreted to fix things, but this excess just ends up storing fat in all the wrong places.

Did you know that sleep also controls hunger? Most people believe that sticking to a diet is about willpower and not eating junk; it's true you need to resist temptation, but hormonal imbalance caused by sleep makes you hungry – it's not just psychological but physiological too! If you sleep less than six hours, the areas of your brain that increase the need for food are triggered and you feel extra hungry – you overeat, beyond your calorie requirement, and look! *Your weight shoots up.*

You need to sleep for at least seven hours a day without interruption. And I don't mean doze or take power naps or even go the entire week without sleeping and then make up for it over the weekend by not getting out of bed. You must sleep from 10-6 at night, because there are certain hormonal responses in your body that take place only at this time – work in tandem with your biological clock so that you stay fit and healthy!

Chapter Three: Step 1: Changing Food Patterns and Fixing Dietary Routines

Food, as we already saw, is the first thing you must change to accommodate weight loss. As the phrase goes, *'you are what you eat'*. And the more junk you eat, the more fat your body accumulates and the more pathetic you feel.

Let's talk more about the kinds of foods you should be eating and the kinds of foods you should be avoiding. Now, a big mistake that people make with their 'diet' plans is expecting to switch over suddenly from eating burgers and fries constantly to only fruits and veggies. While it's what is expected of you during a diet, you can't cut off your addiction that easily without facing withdrawal. And sugar addiction is an actual *physiological* addiction – you must treat it as such.

Instead, think about choosing healthier options as you eat. For instance, if it's a small desert after dinner that you crave, instead of downing that entire brownie and adding to your calories, go in for a single square of melted dark chocolate, interspersed with a ton of nuts like almonds and walnuts. Dark chocolate, taken sparsely, has been proven to help with heart conditions and the nuts give you protein and other nutrients while satisfying your snack craving!

The main nutrients you need to think about when you're focusing on weight loss are proteins, carbohydrates and fats. Before you start your weight loss plan, sit and make a list of all the things you're eating in a day – don't skip over a *single* thing. Even a small mouthful of your favorite soda can make a difference when you're counting calories. Take note of how much carbohydrate you're consuming.

Most people assume that when you want to lose weight, it's about a low-fat diet – that's the biggest misconception. Switching to a low-carb diet is a much better idea. It reduces your appetite and make sure you reduce your calories, but also helps bring blood sugar, pressure and triglycerides down. What happens is that when you consume lower carbs, your body will move into 'ketosis' – instead of glucose from the carbs, it's ketone bodies that will supply energy and ketones kill appetite, thereby helping you lose weight quickly.

Now the issue here is *how* low is a low-carb diet? Different bodies require different amounts; people with an active lifestyle and higher muscle mass can take higher amounts of carbs than those with a sedentary lifestyle. For instance, you'll find that body builders or sprinters take a lot of carbs – they need the energy to maintain the amount of work they do in a day. So figuring out how many carbs you should be eating is, again, individualistic, based on age, sex, body composition, activity levels and rates of body metabolism. But in general, 50-75 grams of carbs in a day should be ideal for weight loss – it gives you just the right amount of carbs you need while helping you lose pounds.

To augment the low-carb intake, you need high intake of protein and fiber. Protein helps to suppress the hunger hormone and instead triggers the satiety hormones in your brain; this means that you lose appetite when you shift to a low-carb, high-protein diet. Automatically, you start eating fewer calories. Another advantage of protein is that it boosts metabolism – people with slower metabolism have a propensity to gain weight, while those with fast metabolism will lose it. So the more protein you consume, the faster your metabolism becomes and you can burn more calories. Proteins also restrict cravings so that snacks go right out the window and help you burn fat instead of muscle mass.

Again, choosing how much protein to consume is dependent on a number of things such as work, age, body composition, etc. Studies show that keeping 30% of your overall calorie intake as protein is best for weight loss, i.e., if you're eating 2000 calories in a day, make sure 600 of those comes straight from protein-foods.

And let me break the biggest weight loss myth – low-fat diets don't work. Not only are they painful to maintain, they actually inhibit fat burning. Your fat cells release certain hormones, such as *adiponectin*, which boost metabolism, increasing the rate at which fat is burnt down. When you go on a low-fat diet, you have lower levels of this hormone, which means you have a propensity to gain weight instead of losing it.

You need to add fats to your diet. Good, satiating fats leave you feeling full, which means a loss of appetite since they trigger production of the satiety hormones. It's the *carbs* you need to avoid, since they mess up your insulin levels and thus, increase fat-mass of your body. Good fats, taken in the place of these carbs, actually help burn your fat, so don't throw them out!

The problem with fatty foods – even good ones – is that it's easy to overindulge. You've to be extremely cautious when you add them to your diet; they *do* add calories and they *are* detrimental to weight loss on a large scale. But if you can get the right quantity in, they'll augment weight loss! Again, the amount to be consumed varies individually, but ballpark it to around 50-100 grams of fat in a day. Replace those regular carbs with both fat and protein and you have the best weight loss!

Now I won't use the word 'dieting' because again, that implies temporary weight management. You need to lose pounds and maintain them, so *lifestyle* change – the issue is most people starve themselves and give up in a few days because it's too hard. When you don't eat at all, or make unhealthy choices such as ignoring all the nutrient groups in favor of only fruits and veggies that are tastelessly made, you're only going to give up easily.

Instead of those big meals, eat smaller, regular meals through the day. Have a big breakfast rich in protein, a mid-morning healthy snack like nuts or fruits, a smaller fiber-rich lunch, a mid-afternoon snack, low-carb dinner and a late-night snack. What you're doing is preempting hunger – if you eat when you're starving, you'll overeat. Also keep in mind that it takes your body 20 minutes to realize that it's full, so you need to stop when you feel about 80% full, or you're actually overeating. And remember – drink plenty of water! It'll help you get rid of the water weight and fill your stomach, thereby ensuring you don't overeat.

Chapter Four: Step 2: Exercising Daily

The second step to any weight loss plan is to start moving. Correcting your food habits can only do so much – you need to burn more and more calories if you want to lose weight. Exercise burns the fat; your body digs into the house of stored fats, burns them and gives you the energy to continue moving through the day. As we saw, exercise releases endorphins, which helps you feel good and happy. People overcome by stress or depression can battle their affliction with exercise – cross that initial barrier and push yourself to exercise and you'll be surprised at how dependent you become on it later!

Exercise also helps you build and strengthen your muscles. In fact, exercising when on a diet is a must because you want to make sure that your body burns the fat and not the muscle. Losing muscle mass is a bad idea – it'll make your body weaker and more susceptible to problems later. When you exercise, though, you'll help your body focus on burning fat and you can strengthen and tighten your muscles.

The question you can then ask is – how much exercise should you do? The issue with most people is that they have unrealistic expectations. You've *never* taken the time to exercise before and suddenly, you want to jump into a 30-minute cardio, which involves running and sprinting – it's no wonder you give up in a day or two! Such heavy-duty exercise requires endurance, which is *built* over time.

Instead, start small and break your weight loss plan into realistic goals. If this is the first time you're exercising, go with a simple brisk walk for 30 minutes in the morning. What you essentially need is a cardio workout – the faster your heart beats, the more fat you burn. The CDC advises that you do a moderate aerobic activity for two and a half hours in a week; that means that doing a 30-minute exercise in the morning each day is a brilliant way to start. Don't do it all at one go; you'll faint and lose energy. Spread it out over the week as 30 minutes each day and make the daily exercise part of your lifestyle; you'll feel more energized during the day!

The next question you ask is – what exercise must you do? Of course, any kind of exercise is necessary, but there are specific types of exercises geared towards specific purposes. For weight loss, cardio is what you need to do. Lifting, for instance, doesn't help in burning fat as much as it does strengthening muscle – so you need to lift and do cardio once you start losing those pounds.

The best exercise for weight loss is walking. It's low impact on your joints, which can be an issue for obese people, and you can do it anywhere, anytime. Of course, if you're looking for accelerated weight loss, that might not be the only answer – you can think of biking, running, swimming, dancing (*Zumba*!) or going to the gym, obviously. Essentially, what you need is a good cardio workout to lose pounds; you can pick and choose what you want to do, but you *must* exercise.

Remember – don't expect too much out of yourself and then give up halfway! Set realistic goals and break it down; being able to run constantly for 20 minutes sounds wonderful, but if you've never ran before, you'll only burnout. Build your endurance levels – if you find that a week of walking briskly is getting easier, up your exercise to jogging and then go for running. Slow but steady progress is the key to losing weight!

Another thing to keep in mind is that you have to exercise in the morning! Going to the gym after work sounds good, but how many times do you actually do it? *You're too tired; you've too much work,* etc. And when you burn calories at the end of the day, you burn only what you've consumed over the day instead of burning stored fat. Work out in the morning and you force your body to burn stored fat – it also energizes you for the whole day, particularly if you exercise out in the open and gulp in that precious, fresh oxygen which is cleanest in the early dawn times. A light evening workout is a good idea, especially if you have trouble sleeping, but don't miss your morning workout!

If you're the kind of person who hates to exercise, then incorporate it into your daily activity instead of making a trip of going to the gym. For instance, instead of specifically going on your morning walk or run, why not try brisk walking to your work? Of course, that does mean that you don't get to shower and end up sweaty and smelly at your job, but you can look for other options! What you need is an active lifestyle instead of a sedentary one; even if you work out daily, exercise without movement in the day is only going to help you *maintain* weight, not lose it. So keep moving through the day; if you're watching TV, get up and pace across the hall during commercial breaks. Or if you're hungry, walk to the nearby store to buy yourself something healthy to eat instead of snacking on junk.

Keep moving – that's the best way to burn calories and lose weight!

Chapter Five: Step 3: Planning Meals and Creating Daily Schedules – Recipes and Exercise Routines

The biggest issue that people miss out on is *planning*. You can't just go on a crash diet – you need to stock your pantry with foods that will augment your weight loss. You need to plan *what* to eat, *when* to eat and you need to work out your routine so that you have time to finish all work and still have space for exercise and a full 7 hours of sleep. So in this chapter, let's look at a sample 7-day routine that will help you get started! Use this plan as a kick-start into a newer lifestyle; remember, you have to *continue* this type of living even after one week or you'll only get all that weight back.

Your schedule should look like this –

6.00 a.m. – Wake up; exercise for a minimum of 30 minutes and breathe in as much fresh oxygen as possible
7.30 a.m. – Breakfast
10.30 a.m. – Mid-morning Snack
12.30 p.m. – Lunch
3.30 p.m. – Mid-afternoon snack
5.30 p.m. – Quick evening workout; can be light
6.30 p.m. – Dinner
9.00 p.m. – Late-night snack
10.30 p.m. – Bedtime

As you can see, we've spread your calorie intake in neat timings over the day so that you can eat in a healthy manner! But what do you eat? It's very simple – you need to consume a big breakfast, with a lot of protein to see you through the day. For lunch, you can add a little fat to your diet and then dinner should be sparse, since you're going to be sleeping after food, adding to fat storage in your body. In between meals you must snack on simple fruits, nuts, vegetables and the like so that you don't overeat at meals. Check out some quick recipes you can make for meals.

Breakfast Foods

Broccoli and Feta Omelet with Toast

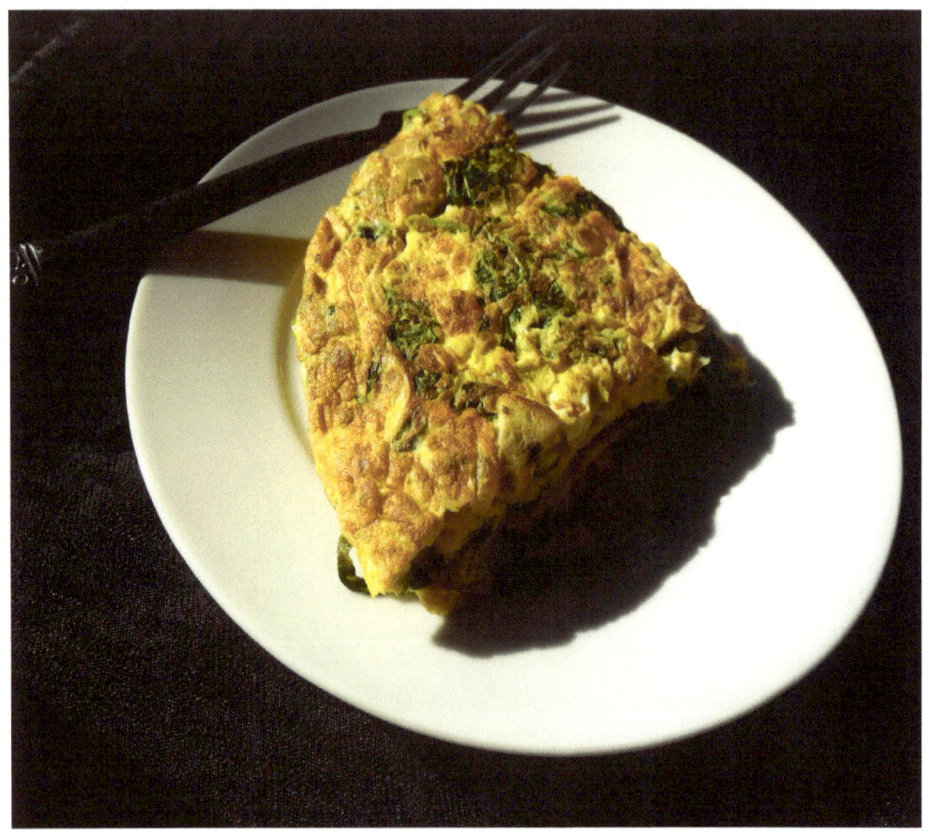

Image courtesy: Pixabay

Serves: 2
Calories per serving: 390
Protein per serving: 23g
Carbs per serving: 35g
Fiber per serving: 6g
Saturated Fat per serving: 6g
Monounsaturated Fat per serving: 5g
Polyunsaturated Fat per serving: 2g

Ingredients:

- 2 cups chopped broccoli

- 4 large eggs, beaten

- 4 tablespoons feta cheese, crumbled

- 4 slices rye bread, toasted

- Cooking spray

Instructions:

Coat pan with cooking spray and cook broccoli over medium heat for 3 minutes. Combine the eggs, feta and dill in a bowl – add this to the pan and cook for another 4 minutes until omelet is cooked on both sides. Serve with the toast.

Banana and Almond Butter Toast

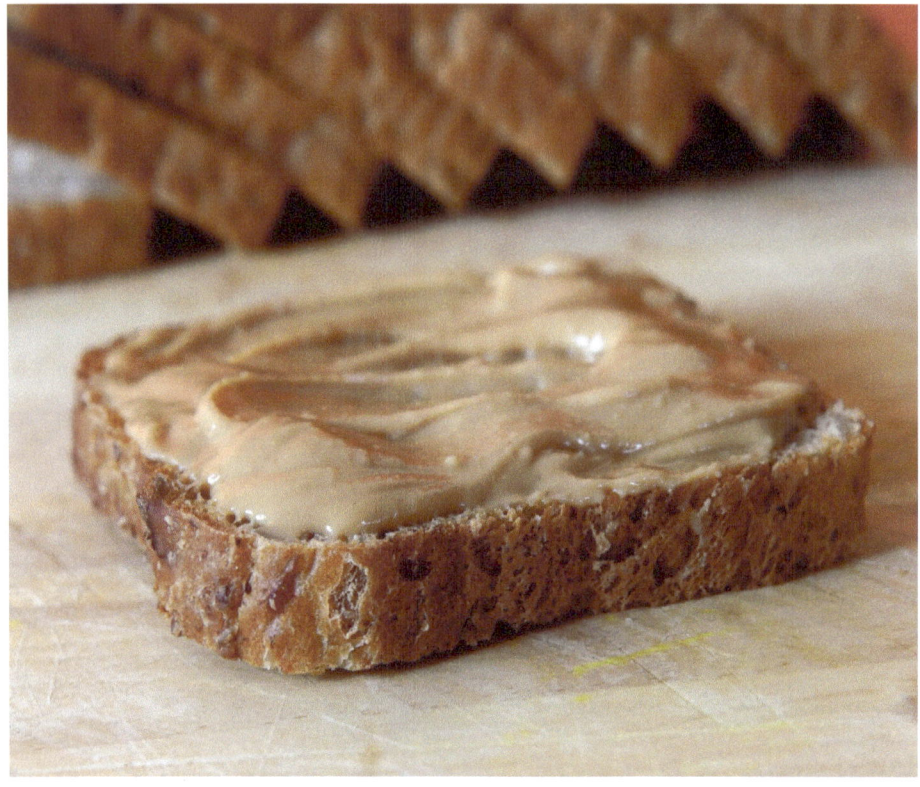

Image courtesy: Pixabay

Serves: 2
Calories per serving: 280
Protein per serving: 6g
Carbs per serving: 44g
Fiber per serving: 5g
Saturated Fat per serving: 1g
Monounsaturated Fat per serving: 7g
Polyunsaturated Fat per serving: 2.5g

Ingredients:

- 2 tablespoons almond butter

- 2 slices rye bread, toasted

- 2 bananas, sliced

Instructions:

Spread the almond butter on the toast and top with banana slices.

Lunch Foods

Curried Egg Salad Sandwich

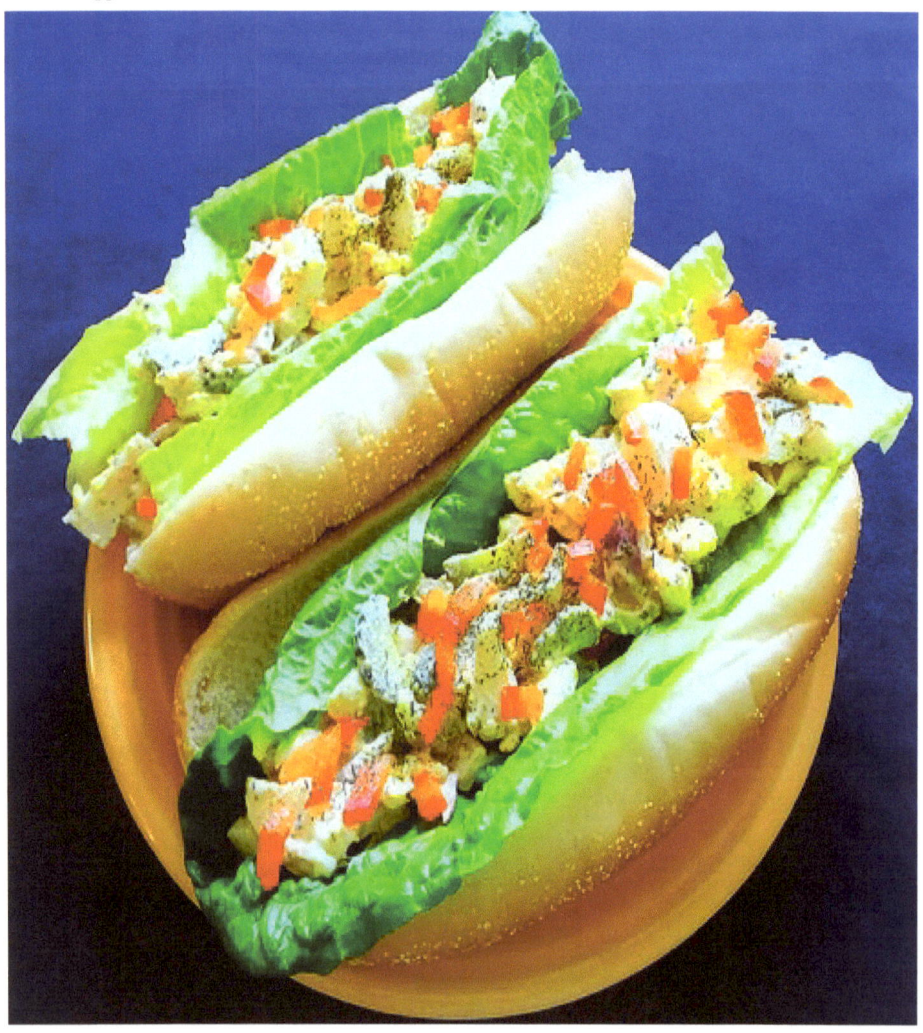

Image courtesy: Flickr

Serves: 2
Calories per serving: 410
Protein per serving: 22g
Carbs per serving: 51g
Fiber per serving: 8g

Saturated Fat per serving: 4g
Monounsaturated Fat per serving: 5g
Polyunsaturated Fat per serving: 2g

Ingredients:

- 4 hard-cooked eggs, chopped

- 4 tablespoons low-fat yogurt

- 4 tablespoons red bell-peppers, chopped

- ½ tablespoon curry powder

- 4 slices rye bread, toasted

- 1 cup spinach

- 2 oranges

- Salt and pepper to taste

Instructions:

Combine the yogurt, the bell pepper and eggs in a bowl and season with the curry powder, salt and pepper. Spread the salad on top of the rye bread, top with the spinach and then serve with the orange on the side.

BBQ Turkey Burgers

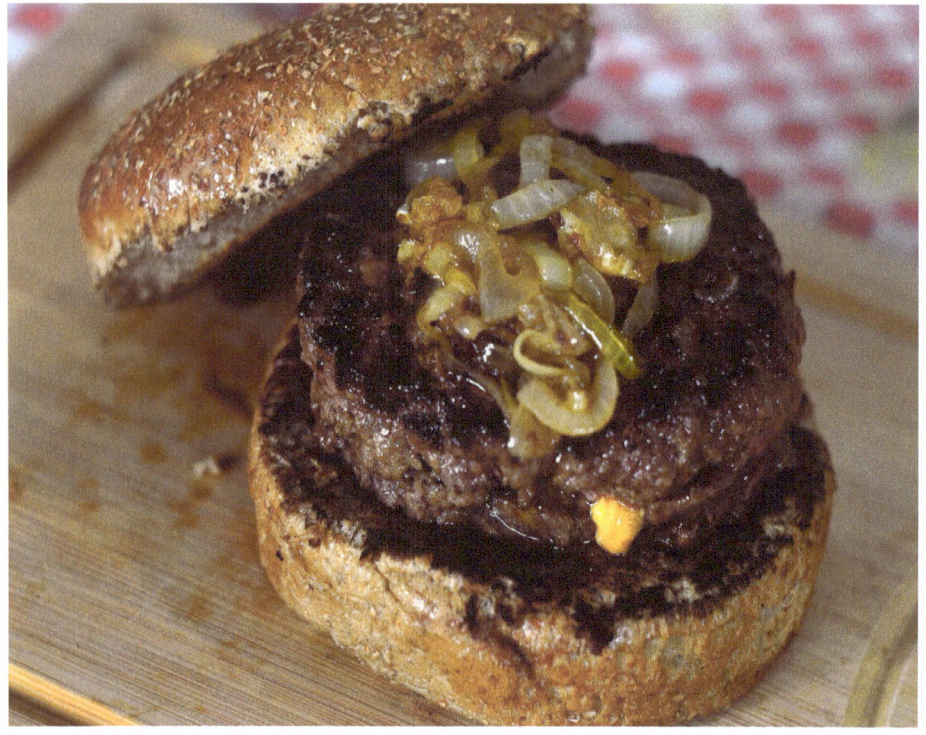

Image courtesy: Pixabay

Serves: 2

Calories per serving: 324
Protein per serving: 28g
Carbs per serving: 28g
Fiber per serving: 1g
Saturated Fat per serving: 2.7g
Monounsaturated Fat per serving: 3.3g
Polyunsaturated Fat per serving: 3.9g

Ingredients:
- ½ pound ground dark-meat turkey

- ½ garlic clove, minced

- ¼ spoon paprika

- 1/8 spoon cumin, ground

- 2 slices sweet onion, grilled

- 1/8 cup barbecue sauce

- 2 sesame seed buns, roasted

- Salt and pepper

Instructions:

Mix the turkey, garlic, cumin and paprika together in a bowl; now flatten it into two small patties and season with salt/pepper. Heat your grill to medium heat and cook the patties for about 7 minutes each, until fully cooked on both sides. Top with onions and sauce and serve.

Dinner Foods

Middle Eastern Rice Salad

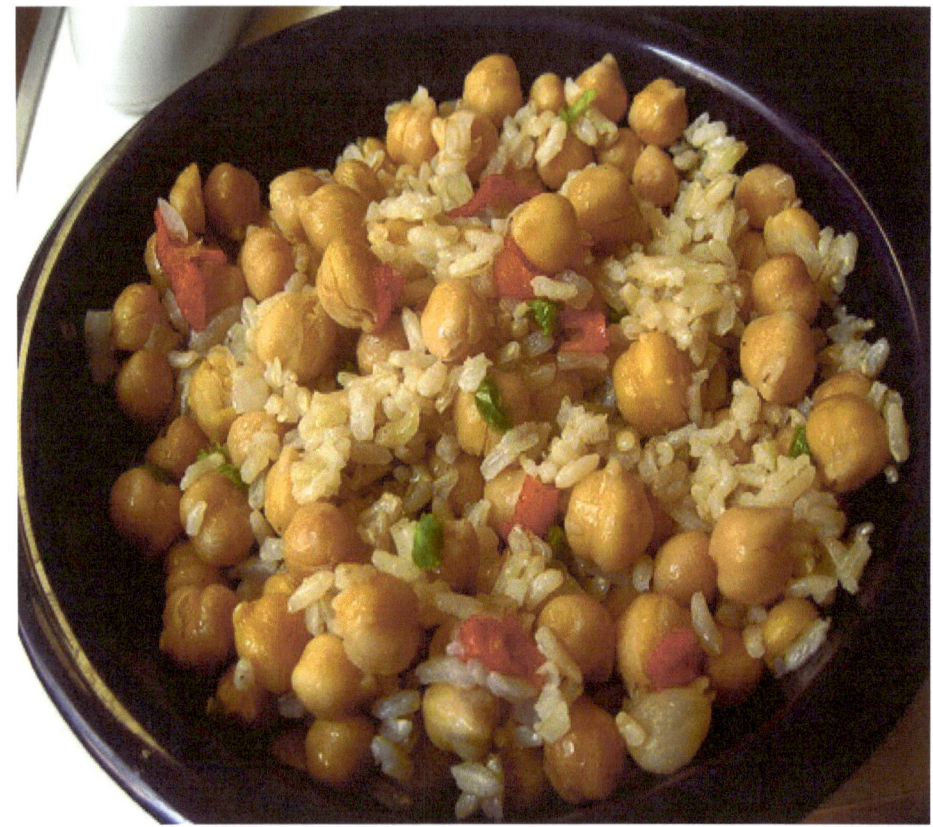

Image courtesy: Flickr

Serves: 2
Calories per serving: 380
Protein per serving: 8g
Carbs per serving: 67g
Fiber per serving: 8g
Saturated Fat per serving: 1g
Monounsaturated Fat per serving: 5.5g
Polyunsaturated Fat per serving: 1g

Ingredients:

- 1 tablespoon olive oil
- ½ cup sweet onion, thinly sliced
- ½ 16-ounce can chickpeas, drained and rinsed
- ¼ spoon cumin, ground
- 1 ½ cups brown rice
- ¼ cup pitted dates
- 1/8 cup mint, chopped
- 1/8 cup parsley, chopped
- Salt and pepper

Instructions:

Heat some oil over a medium flame and cook the onions until it turns brown. Remove from heat and stir in the chickpeas. Season with cumin and salt/pepper; in a bowl, combine this mixture with rice, dates, mint and the parsley. Toss well and serve.

Spicy Southwestern Black-Bean Chili

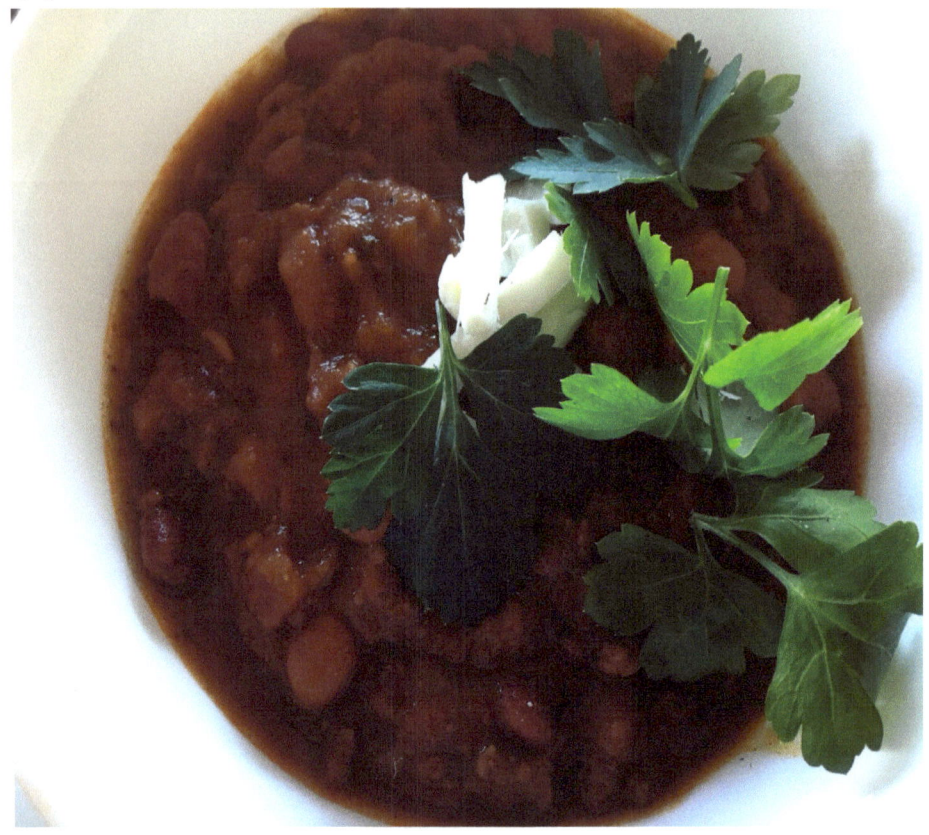

Image courtesy: Pixabay

Serves: 2
Calories per serving: 391
Protein per serving: 17g
Carbs per serving: 57g
Fiber per serving: 13g
Saturated Fat per serving: 4g
Monounsaturated Fat per serving: 5g
Polyunsaturated Fat per serving: 1g

Ingredients:

- 1 tablespoon olive oil

- ¾ cup onion, chopped

- ½ cup jalapenos, chopped/seeded

- ½ garlic clove, chopped

- 1 tablespoon chili powder

- ½ tablespoon cumin, ground

- 2 32-ounce boxes boxed roasted red pepper and tomato soup

- 1 15.5-ounce can black-bean, rinsed/drained

- 1/8 cup low-fat sour-cream

- 1/8 cup cilantro, chopped

Instructions:

Heat some oil over a medium flame and cook onions and jalapenos until they soften. Stir garlic, chili powder, cumin and cook for a minute, before stirring the back-beans in. simmer this for 5 minutes before adding chopped cilantro. Now ladle into soup bowls and top with 1 tablespoon of sour cream and season with salt and pepper as required.

Snacks

Honey Grapefruit with Banana

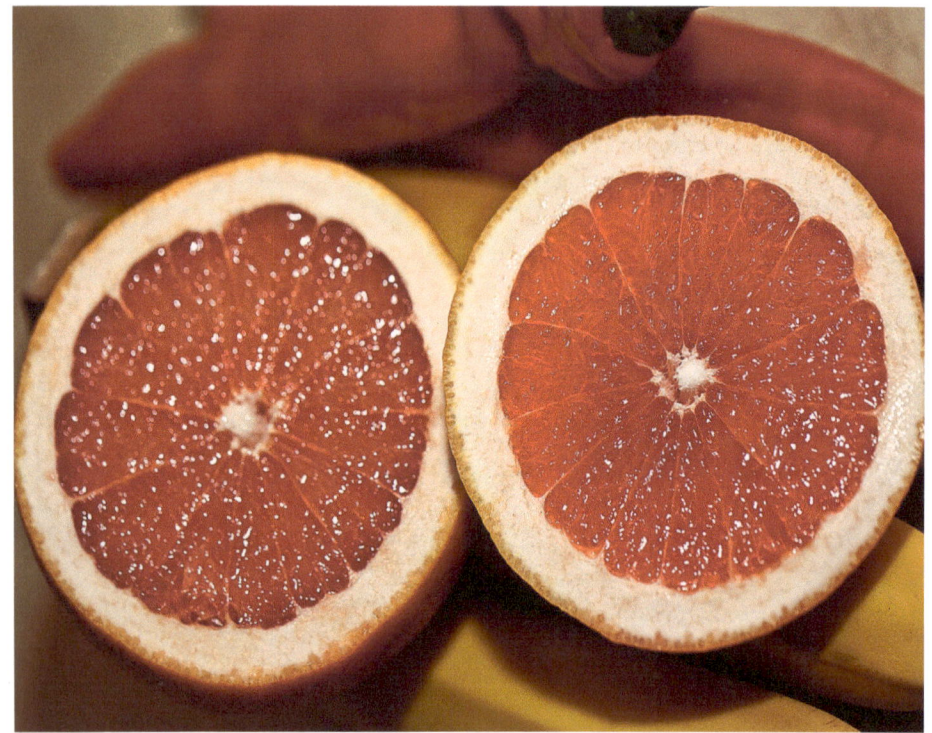

Image courtesy: Pixabay

Serves: 6
Calories per serving: 122
Protein per serving: 1.5g
Carbs per serving: 31.3g
Fiber per serving: 3.4g
Saturated Fat per serving: 0.1g
Monounsaturated Fat per serving: 0g
Polyunsaturated Fat per serving: 0g

Ingredients:
- 4 cups red grapefruit sections

- 2 bananas, sliced

- 2 tablespoons mint, chopped

- 2 tablespoons honey

Instructions:

Drain the grapefruit sections, reserving ¼ the juice. Throw them in with the rest of the ingredients in a bowl and toss to mix. Serve.

Dark Chocolate and Oat Clusters

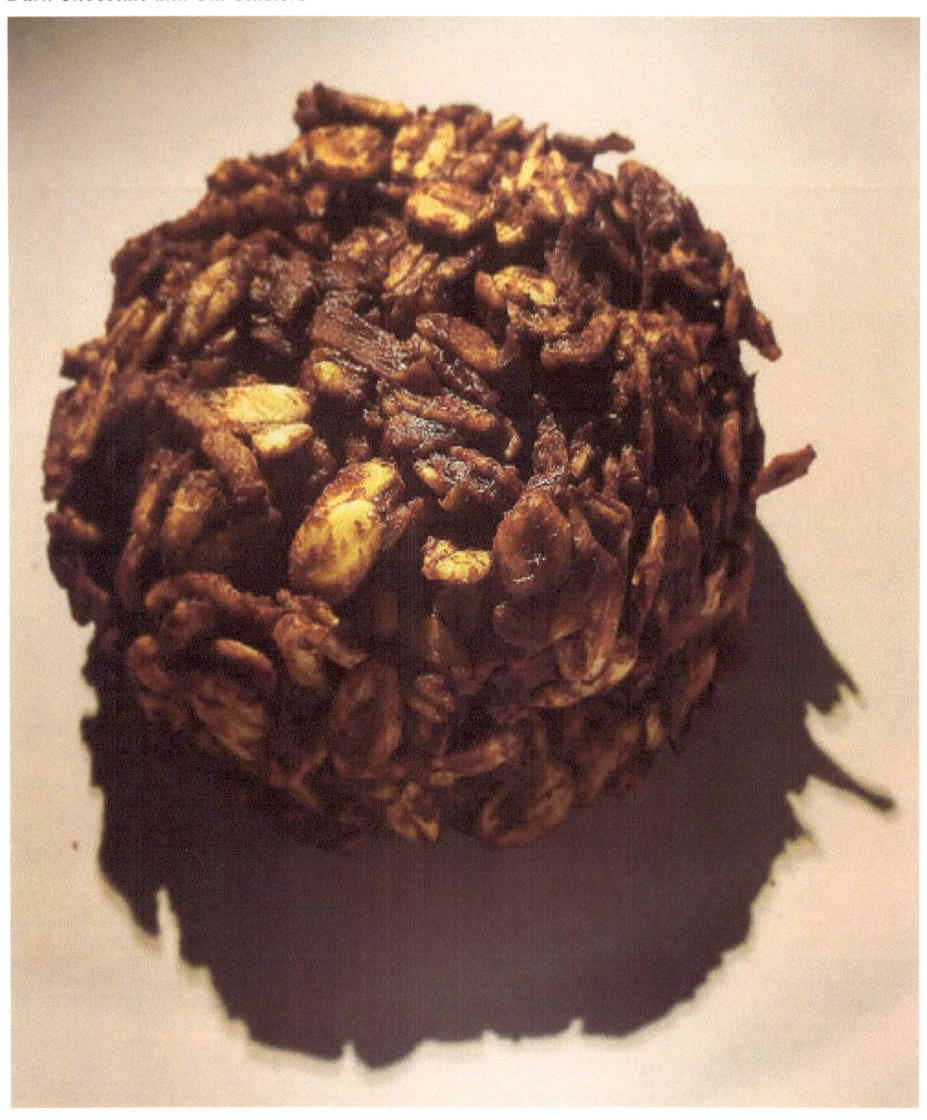

Image courtesy: Flickr

Serves: 2
Calories per serving: 160
Protein per serving: 5g
Carbs per serving: 19g

Fiber per serving: 3g
Saturated Fat per serving: 3g
Monounsaturated Fat per serving: 3.5g
Polyunsaturated Fat per serving: 1.5g

Ingredients:
- 1 tablespoon peanut butter

- 1 tablespoon low-fat milk

- 1/8 cup dark chocolate chips

- 1/3 cup old-fashioned rolled oats

Instructions:
Heat the peanut butter, chocolate chips and milk over low heat until chips melt. Stir in oats and remove from heat. Use a spoon to drop ball-shaped portion on to wax paper-lined baking sheet and refrigerate for 10 minutes.

Smoothies to Drink

Spiced Green Tea Smoothie

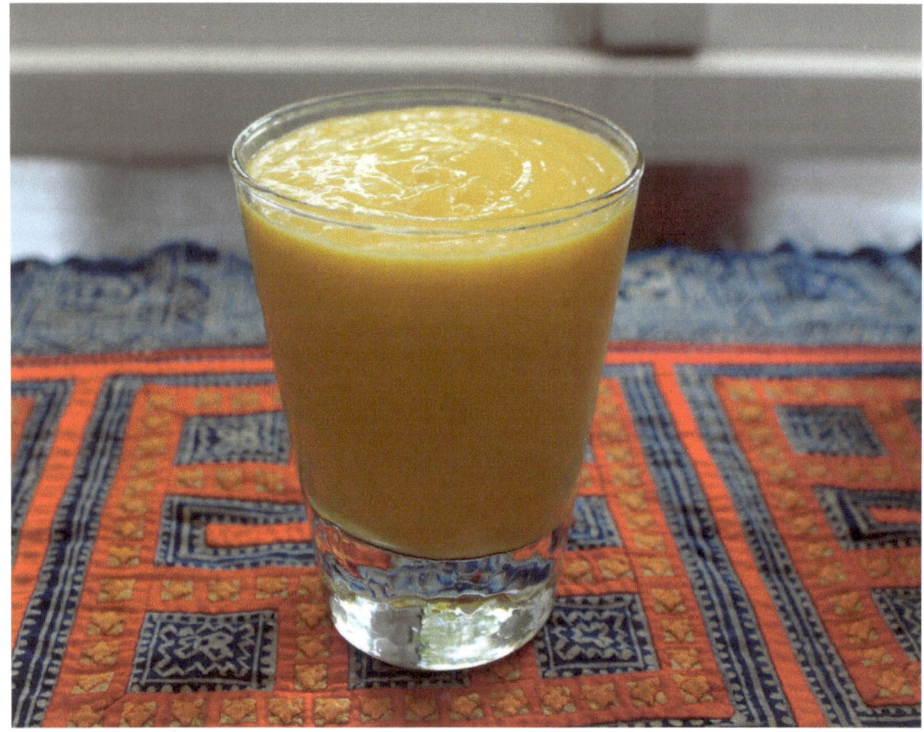

Image courtesy: Flickr

Serves: 1
Calories per serving: 82
Protein per serving: 1g
Carbs per serving: 21g
Fiber per serving: 3g
Saturated Fat per serving: 0g
Monounsaturated Fat per serving: 0g
Polyunsaturated Fat per serving: 0g

Ingredients:

- 1/3 cup strong green-tea, chilled

- 1/8 spoon cayenne pepper

- ½ lemon's juice

- 1 teaspoon agave nectar

- ½ pear, skin-on cut slices

- 1 tablespoon low-fat yogurt

- 3-4 ice-cubes

Instructions:
Throw it altogether in a blender and make creamy mixture – drink cold!

Spinach and Avocado Smoothie

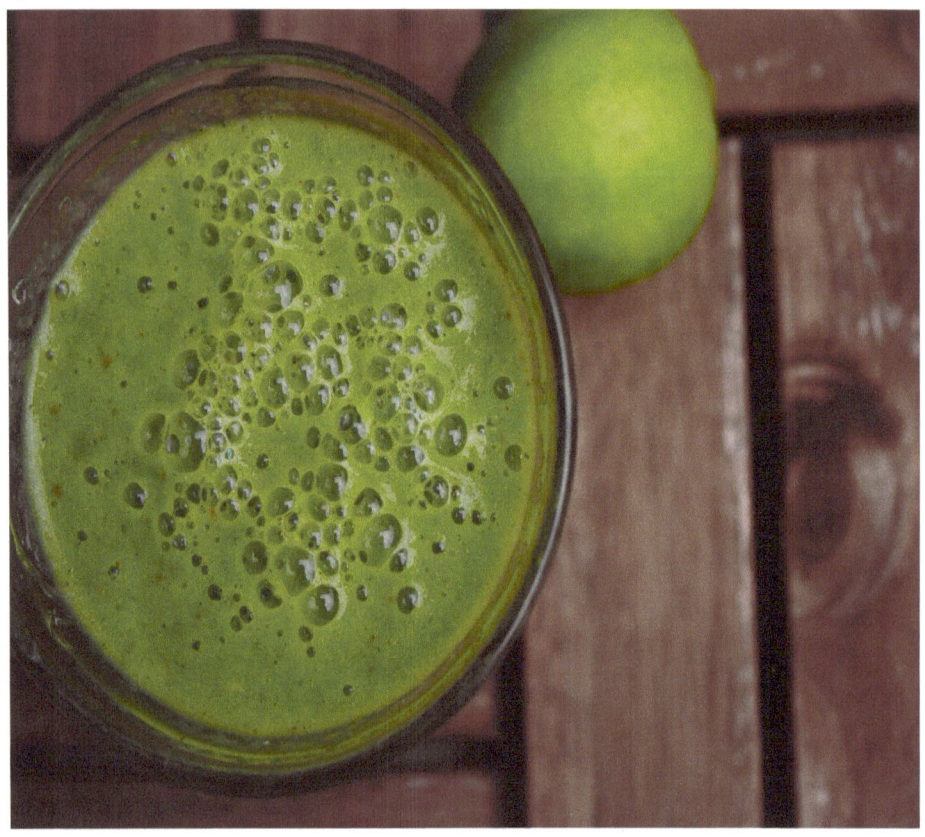

Image courtesy: Flickr

Serves: 1
Calories per serving: 338
Protein per serving: 7.7g
Carbs per serving: 29.2g
Fiber per serving: 3g
Saturated Fat per serving: 6g
Monounsaturated Fat per serving: 0g
Polyunsaturated Fat per serving: 0g

Ingredients:

- ½ avocado, pitted

- ½ cup spinach

- ½ banana

- ½ teaspoon peanut butter

- ½ cup milk

- 3-4 ice-cubes

Instructions:
Throw it altogether in a blender and make creamy mixture.

Banana Cream Pie

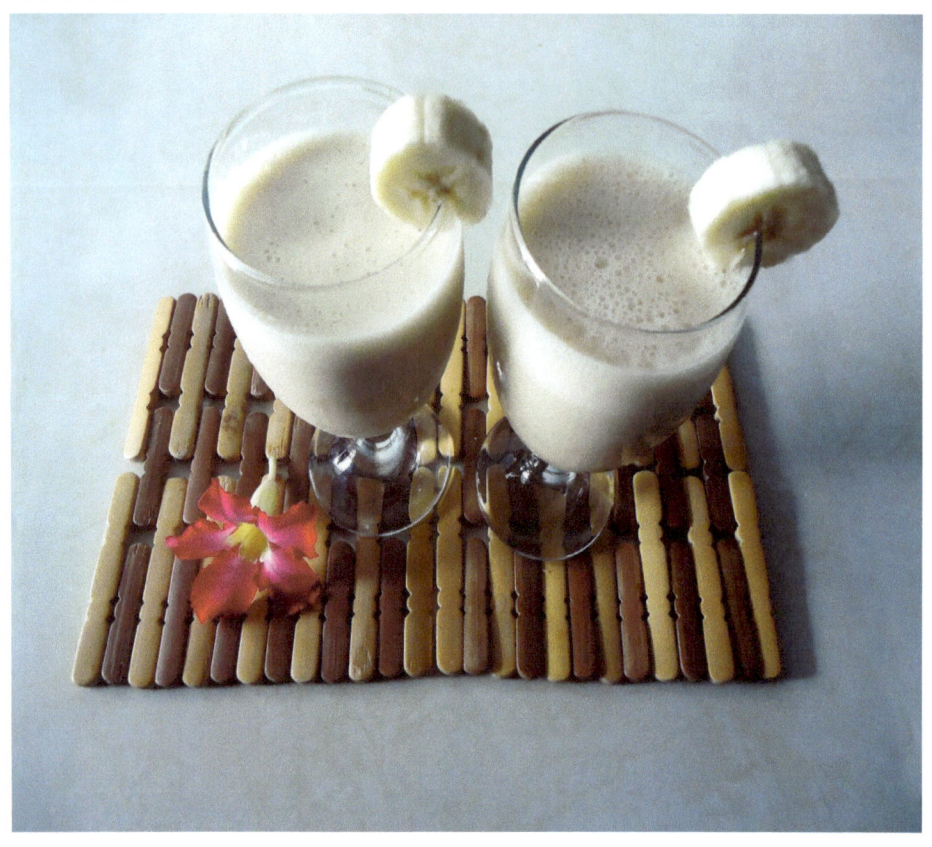

Image courtesy: Flickr

Serves: 1
Calories per serving: 216
Protein per serving: 9.8g
Carbs per serving: 39.3g
Fiber per serving: 1.9g
Saturated Fat per serving: 1.5g
Monounsaturated Fat per serving: 0.8g
Polyunsaturated Fat per serving: 0.3g

Ingredients:
- ½ banana, frozen

- ½ cup low-fat yogurt

- ¼ spoon vanilla extract

- 1 tablespoon honey

- 1/8 cup milk

- 3-4 ice-cubes

- Graham cracker crumbs, crushed

Instructions:
Throw it altogether in a blender and make creamy mixture. Sprinkle the cracker crumbs on top to garnish.

See how many *tasty* recipes you can make? Once you get the hang of picking the right kind of foods, you can play around and make your own meal-plans that'll help you lose weight! Plan your meals a week in advance and stock your pantry – make sure you buy foods that are rich in protein, with less carbs!

Tips to remember while grocery shopping is to never shop hungry, shop with a list and stick to the outer aisles of the store, where the fresh fruits and veggies are stored. Throw out all starchy, sugary foods and replace with healthy items – once you restock your pantry, you can create new recipes with the healthier options you have!

The next thing, of course, is exercise. As we said, weight loss requires consistent exercise, so here are some things you can try out. Remember, the idea is to do *cardio*. If you don't like working out in gyms, you can exercise at home!

Cardio

You *need* to do a 30-minute cardio every day. You can walk, run or do aerobics or Zumba at home – you don't have to go to the gym. But you need to get moving and make sure you build endurance as well as muscle; lifting weights is a good idea to strengthen and tighten muscles. When you go to the gym, you usually do a full routine that starts with a warm-up session, has a 30-minute cardio workout and then ends with another quick stretch session. But you don't need to go to the gym to do that; you can do it at home!

Here is a sample exercise routine you can try –

Full-body Warm-Up Sessions

Warming up before you do any kind of exercise is vital. Your body, which has been at a state of rest so far, needs to wake up – if you jump straight into hardcore exercise, you could pull a muscle. As with anything, you need to work your way up to hard workouts, which is why we always do warm-up exercises. Even if you are simply going for a 30-minute walk around the neighborhood, make sure you do a few stretches to get your blood pumping and then go! Here is a list of warm-up exercises you can try at home for this sample workout routine –

- March-in-place – As the name suggests, you have to stand in one place and then march. Make sure your past is fast; bring your left elbow to the front as your right knee comes up. Keep this up for 60 seconds and breathe slowly and steadily throughout the entire minute.

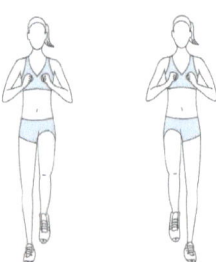

Source: http://www.spotebi.com/wp-content/uploads/2015/02/march-in-place-exercise-illustration.jpg

- Jumping Rope – Remember playing rope as a kid? That's one brilliant exercise that you can restart again! Jump with the balls of your feet and make sure you keep your knees slightly bent. Do this for another 60 seconds. Remember to turn the rope only with your wrists – don't use your entire arms!

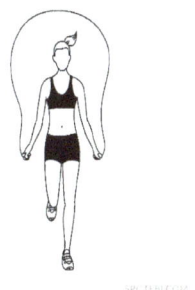

- Jumping Jacks – Stand straight with your hands by your sides and then jump, bringing both hands together above your head and your feet spreading. Jump a second time to bring yourself back to original position. Do this for another 60 seconds; make sure to keep your knees bent and jump with the balls of your feet.

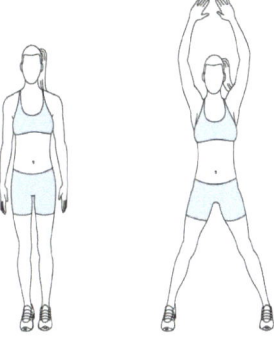

- Butt Kicks – Stand straight with your feet at shoulder-width distance. Start kicking your feet up and back, until your heels touch your glutes. Pump your right arm in sync with your left leg and vice versa. Keep this up for the next 60 seconds. Remember to keep your shoulders back, your arms close to your torso and your elbows bent at 90 degree.

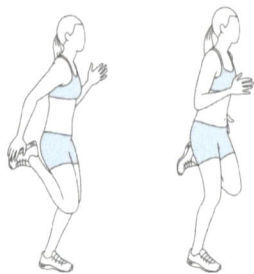

Source: http://www.spotebi.com/wp-content/uploads/2015/01/butt-kicks-exercise-illustration.jpg

- High Kicks – Stand straight with your feet at shoulder-width distance. Now lift one leg as fast as you can and kick in front of you; return to standing position and do the same with the other leg. Alternate for the next 60 seconds. Keep your knee straight and breathe out as you kick.

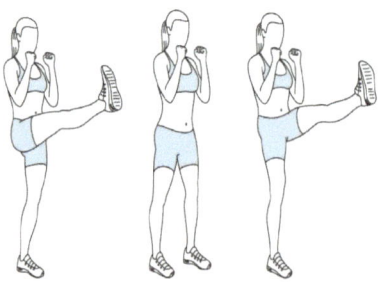

Source:http://www.spotebi.com/wp-content/uploads/2015/01/high-kicks-exercise-illustration.jpg?14c30d

- Alternating Side-Lunges – Stand straight with your feet at hip-width distance. Now, step to your side with the left leg and touch your left foot with your right hand. Come back to the starting position and repeat the same with the opposite side. Alternate this way for the next 60 seconds.

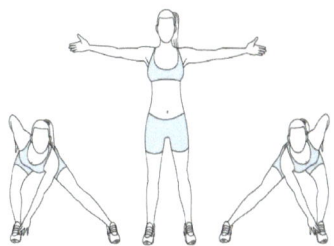

- Big Arm-Circles – Stand straight with your feet at shoulder-width distance. Now, raise your arms without bending the elbows and slowly rotate them forward, making big circles. Do 60 seconds of forward rotations and then do another 60 seconds of backwards rotation. Keep your back straight and don't bend your elbows.

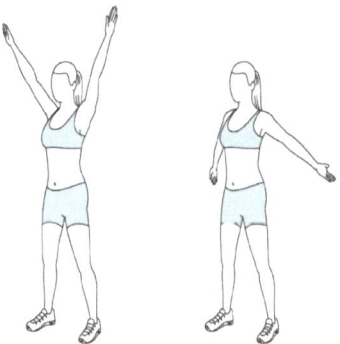

- Hip Circles – Stand straight with your feet a bit wider than shoulder-width; put your hands on your hips and bend your knees slightly. Now, slowly rotate hips and make big circles. Do 60 seconds of this before switching directions to do another 60 seconds of the reverse side. Remember to keep your hips level with the floor.

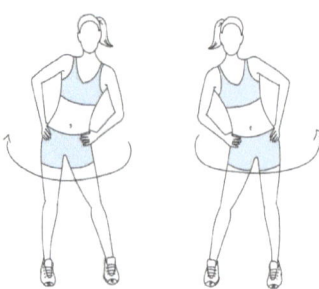

Source: http://www.spotebi.com/wp-content/uploads/2015/01/hip-circles-exercise-illustration.jpg

These are some of the most basic warm-up exercises. Once you do these, you can then start your cardio of 30 minutes.

30-Minute Workout

You can do whatever you like that gets your heart pumping, from walking to Zumba, but here are some quick circuit exercises that will burn calories at home –

- Reverse Lunges and Shoulder Presses – Stand with your feet at shoulder-width distance and hold the dumbbells at shoulder level. Step back with your left leg and then lunge. When you stand up again, push up the dumbbells and lift your left knee to the waist-level. Do this for the next 30 seconds and switch to your right leg to do another 30 seconds of the same.

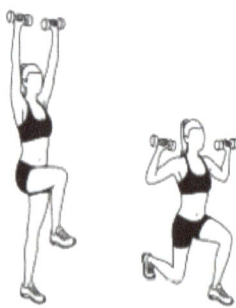

Source: http://www.spotebi.com/workout-routines/30-minute-full-body-fat-burning-workout/

- Alternating Dumbbell Swing – Hold a dumbbell in your left hand. Now squat, bringing the dumbbell between your legs. Stand up and then swing it to your chest and switch hands and repeat the same with your right hand. Do this for the next 60 seconds.

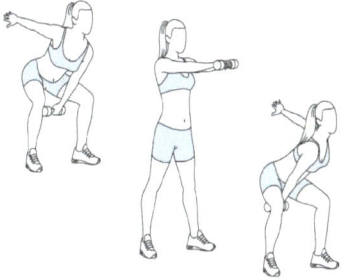

Source:http://www.spotebi.com/wp-content/uploads/2016/04/alternating-dumbbell-swing-exercise-illustration-spotebi.jpg

- Chest Press with Legs – Lie down on your back and raise your legs up to 45 degrees. Push the dumbbells to the ceiling; your palms must face your legs and your shoulders have to be straight, with your arms directly above them. Do this for the next 60 seconds.

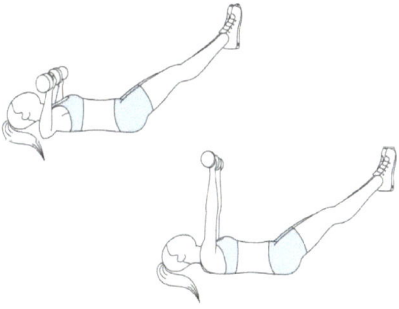

Source: http://www.spotebi.com/wp-content/uploads/2016/02/chest-press-with-legs-extended-exercise-illustration-spotebi.jpg

- Curtsy Lunge Kick – Stand with the dumbbell in your left hand and take a big step back with your right leg. Cross it behind the left and then lunge. When you stand up, kick your right leg out to the side; raise the dumbbell to shoulder height. Do this for the next 30 seconds and then switch to the other side for another 30 seconds.

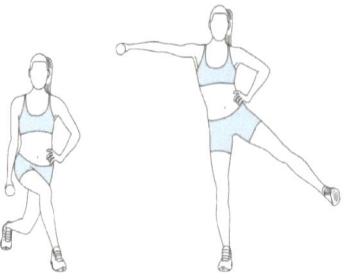

Source:http://www.spotebi.com/wp-content/uploads/2016/02/curtsy-lunge-side-kick-lateral-raise-exercise-illustration-spotebi.jpg

- Balance Chop – Hold the dumbbell with both your hands and rotate your entire torso to the right. Raise the dumbbell above your head and lift your left knee up as your rotate and then when you rotate back, bring it down diagonally to the opposite side. Repeat the other side as well and alternate for 60 seconds.

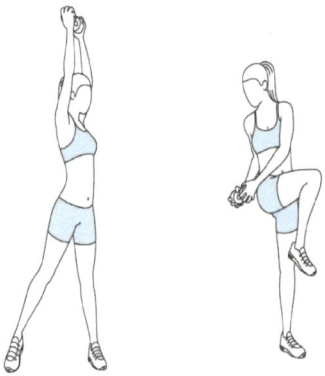

Source:http://www.spotebi.com/wp-content/uploads/2016/06/balance-chop-exercise-illustration-spotebi.jpg

- Plank Straight-Arm Kickback – Get into the plank position – your wrists are under your shoulders and your feet at hip-width distance. Now, lift up on arm back, keeping it straight. Come to plank position and switch sides. Alternate for 60 seconds.

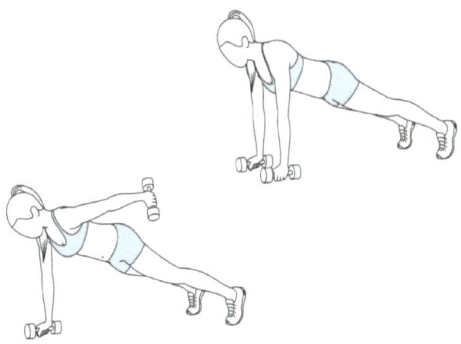

- Wood Chop – Stand with feet and shoulder-width distance, holding dumbbell with both hands. Rotate your torso to the left and bring your dumbbell above your left shoulder. Squat as you turn your torso to the right and bring the dumbbell across your body in a diagonal manner before you come back to starting position. Do this for 30 seconds before switching to the other side for another 30 seconds.

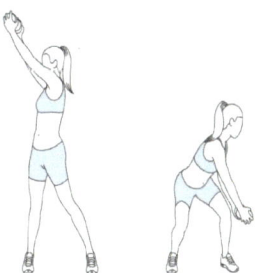

- Split Squat Curl – Stand in a split leg position; keep one leg in the front and the other in the back. Flex your knees and lower your hips – squeeze your biceps as you curl. Lower your arms and then stand up. Do this for 30 seconds before switching legs to complete another 30 seconds.

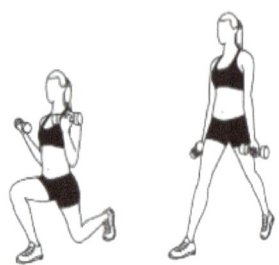

Source: http://www.spotebi.com/workout-routines/30-minute-full-body-fat-burning-workout/

- Thrusters – Hold your dumbbells just in front of your shoulders and squat. When you stand up, raise your arms above your head. Do this for 60 seconds.

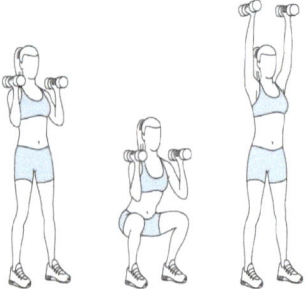

Source:http://www.spotebi.com/wp-content/uploads/2015/04/dumbbell-thrusters-exercise-illustration.jpg

- Plank Rotations – Get into the plank position – your wrists are under your shoulders and your feet at hip-width distance. Twist your torso and then lift your right hand towards the ceiling and look up. Bring it back down and repeat with left hand. Alternate for 60 seconds.

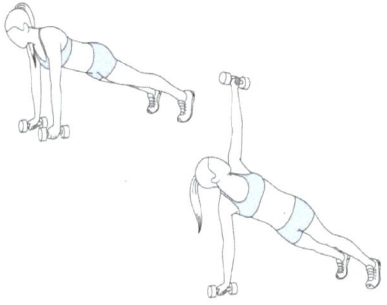

As you can see, when you complete one circuit of these exercises, you'd have finished a 10-minute workout. Complete 3 sets and take a 60-second breathing gap between each – you've finished a 30-minute workout at home! Now you must finish with your stretches again.

Full-Body End-Workout Stretches

Once you finish your workout, you can't just stop. You've built up the momentum, you need to slow it down before you finish! You have to stretch again to end – it'll cool your body down, help you relax and ensure you don't cramp your muscles. Here are some quick stretches you can try –

- Child's Pose – Get onto your hands and knees and then sit on your heels. Separate your knees and lay your upper body down with your arms stretched in front of you. Rest your head on the floor. Breathe slowly and hold for 30 seconds.

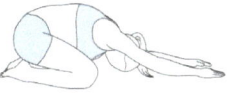

- Abs Stretch – Lie face down, with arms in push-up position. Keep your arms straight and lift up your torso. Hold for 30 seconds.

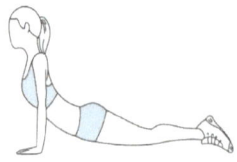

Source: http://www.spotebi.com/wp-content/uploads/2014/11/ab-stretch-exercise-illustration.jpg

- Standing Forward Bend – Stand straight; keep your knees straight and bend at the hips. Grab the back of your ankles. Hold for 30 seconds.

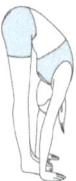

Source:http://www.spotebi.com/wp-content/uploads/2016/01/standing-forward-bend-pose-uttanasana.jpg

- Quad Stretch – Stand straight; shift your weight to your right leg as you lift your left up behind your back. Pull it forward towards your butt until you feel the stretch in your quads. Hold for 30 seconds and then shift to other leg and repeat for another 30 seconds.

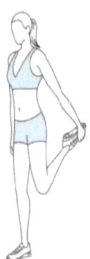

Source: http://www.spotebi.com/wp-content/uploads/2015/03/quad-stretch-exercise-illustration.jpg

These are just a few of the stretches you can start with; be sure to cool your body down, no matter what kind of cardio you do!

With that, you've completed a whole exercise routine! Do this without fail every single day for the next week – you will definitely start losing pounds! Remember, you must continue to exercise every day, no matter what happens; maintaining and sustaining weight loss is dependent on changing lifestyle and regularly exercising!

But remember, exercise and food alone are not enough! The idea is to change your *whole* lifestyle and that includes sleeping well, resting and relaxing, making sure you drink plenty of water, etc.! You *have* to sleep for at least 7 hours and you *have* to do it at nighttime. You *must* drink 8 glasses of water – minimum – in a day. Take a day off to rest and recuperate; weight loss is as much about being happy as it is about 'dieting' and exercising.

Conclusion

Thank you again for downloading this book!

I hope this book was able to help you identify what weight loss is and why you need to focus on it. Sustained weight loss is a matter of time and patience, so start today and don't give up! The next step is to start making those lifestyle changes that will help you shed pounds permanently – change your food patterns, start exercising, get enough sleep and see what a difference that makes to your life!

Finally, if you enjoyed this book, then I'd like to ask you for a favor, would you be kind enough to leave a review for this book on Amazon? It'd be greatly appreciated!

Click here to leave a review for this book on Amazon!

https://www.amazon.com/WEIGHT-LOSS-Practical-Step-Step-ebook/dp/B01MR9SY33/ref=sr_1_1?s=digital-text&ie=UTF8&qid=1488883683&sr=1-1&keywords=weight+loss

Thank you and good luck!

www.ingramcontent.com/pod-product-compliance
Lightning Source LLC
Chambersburg PA
CBHW040326010626
45792CB00024B/2174